Osteoporosis Diet Cookbook for Seniors

Eat Well and Keep Your Bones Strong

Dr Olivia Tastewell

Copyright © 2024 by Dr Olivia Tastewell

Kindly scan the barcode below to reach out to the author and have access to more of our books.

TABLE OF CONTENTS

Introduction

HAVE YOU EVER WONDERED WHAT YOUR bones are made of? You might think they are solid and unchanging, like rocks or metal. But the truth is, your bones are living tissues that constantly break down and rebuild themselves throughout your life. They are composed of minerals, proteins, and cells that work together to give you strength, stability, and flexibility.

But as you age, your bones can become weaker and more prone to fractures. This condition is called osteoporosis, and it affects millions of seniors around the world. Osteoporosis can cause pain, disability, and loss of independence. It can also increase your risk of other health problems, such as heart disease, diabetes, and depression.

You may feel helpless and hopeless when faced with osteoporosis.

You may think there is nothing you can do to prevent or treat it. You may think you have to give up your favorite foods and activities. You may think you have to accept a lower quality of life. However, you are not alone, nor are you powerless. There is a lot you can do to protect your bones and improve your health. One of the most important things you can do is to eat well. Eating well means choosing foods that provide the nutrients your bones need, such as calcium, vitamin D, protein, and antioxidants. It also means avoiding foods that can harm your bones, such as excess salt, sugar, caffeine, and alcohol. It also means enjoying a variety of foods that are delicious, satisfying, and easy to prepare. That's why I created this cookbook for you. In this book, you will find 20 recipes for breakfast, lunch, and dinner that are specially designed for seniors with osteoporosis. These recipes are based on the latest scientific research and recommendations from experts in the field of nutrition and bone health. They are also inspired by my personal experience as a senior who has been living with osteoporosis for over a decade. I know how hard it can be to change your eating habits and lifestyle. I know how frustrating it can be to deal with the pain and limitations of osteoporosis. I know how scary it can be to face the future with uncertainty and fear.

But I also know how rewarding it can be to take charge of your health and happiness. I know how empowering it can be to learn new skills and discover new flavors. I know how joyful it can be to share your food and stories with your loved ones. That's why I want to share this cookbook with you. I want to show you that you can eat well and keep your bones strong. I want to show you that you can still enjoy your food and your life. I want to show you that you can overcome osteoporosis and thrive as a senior.

So, are you ready to join me on this journey? Are you ready to learn more about osteoporosis and nutrition? Are you ready to try some delicious and nutritious recipes? Are you ready to eat well and keep your bones strong?

If you are, then turn the page, and let's get started!

Breakfast Recipes

Citrus Berry Smoothie with Yogurt

Ingredients:

- 1 cup plain Greek yogurt (low-fat or unsweetened almond milk alternative)
- 1/2 cup mixed frozen berries
- 1/2 orange, peeled and segmented
- 1/4 cup orange juice
- 1/2 banana
- 1 tablespoon chia seeds
- Pinch of ground cinnamon (optional)

Nutritional Information (per serving):

- Calories: 300
- Fat: 5g (1g saturated)
- Carbs: 40g (5g fiber)
- Protein: 20g
- Calcium: 300mg (30% DV)

Cooking Time: 5 minutes

Serving Size: 1 large glass

Instructions:

1. Put everything in a blender and blend until it's smooth and creamy.
2. Pour into a glass and enjoy!

Label: High in protein and calcium, packed with antioxidants, customizable with different fruits and yogurt, gluten-free option (almond milk).

Greek Yogurt Parfait with Berries and Almonds

Ingredients:

- 1 cup plain Greek yogurt (low-fat or unsweetened almond milk alternative)
- 1/2 cup mixed fresh berries
- 1/4 cup sliced almonds
- 1/4 cup granola (optional)
- Drizzle of honey or maple syrup (optional)

Nutritional Information (per serving):

- Calories: 350
- Fat: 10g (2g saturated)
- Carbs: 35g (5g fiber)
- Protein: 25g
- Calcium: 300mg (30% DV)

Cooking Time: 5 minutes

Serving Size: 1 parfait glass or bowl

Instructions:

1. Layer yogurt, berries, almonds, and granola (if using) in a parfait glass or bowl.
2. Drizzle with honey or maple syrup if desired.

Label: Rich in protein and calcium, a good source of healthy fats and fiber, versatile with different toppings, gluten-free option (omit granola).

Oatmeal with Almond Milk and Chia Seeds

Ingredients:

- 1/2 cup rolled oats
- 1 cup unsweetened almond milk (low-fat milk option)
- 1/4 cup water
- 1 tablespoon chia seeds
- 1/4 teaspoon vanilla extract
- Pinch of cinnamon
- Fresh fruit (optional)

Nutritional Information (per serving):

- Calories: 250
- Fat: 5g (1g saturated)
- Carbs: 40g (5g fiber)
- Protein: 5g
- Calcium: 100mg (10% DV)

Cooking Time: 10 minutes

Serving Size: 1 bowl

Instructions:

1. Combine oats, almond milk, water, chia seeds, vanilla extract, and cinnamon in a saucepan.
2. Bring to a boil, then reduce heat and simmer for 5-7 minutes, stirring occasionally, until oats are cooked through and chia seeds have plumped.
3. Serve warm with fresh fruit if desired.

Label: High in fiber and whole grains, good source of healthy fats, customizable with different spices and toppings, vegan option (use plant-based milk).

Whole Wheat Blueberry Pancakes

Ingredients:

- 1 cup whole wheat flour
- 1 1/2 teaspoons baking powder
- 1/4 teaspoon salt
- 1 cup milk (low-fat or unsweetened almond milk option)
- 1 egg
- 1 tablespoon honey
- 1/4 cup blueberries
- Olive oil for greasing pan

Nutritional Information (per serving):

- Calories: 250
- Fat: 5g (1g saturated)
- Carbs: 40g (4g fiber)
- Protein: 8g
- Calcium: 100mg (10% DV)

Cooking Time: 15 minutes

Serving size: 2

Instructions:

1. In a large bowl, whisk together dry ingredients (flour, baking powder, and salt).
2. In a separate bowl, whisk together milk, egg, and honey.
3. Pour the wet ingredients into the dry ingredients and stir until just combined, leaving some lumps for a fluffy texture. Gently fold in blueberries.
4. Warm up a pan with a bit of oil on it over medium heat.
5. Pour 1/4 cup batter per pancake and cook for 2-3 minutes per side, or until golden brown and bubbles appear on the surface.
6. Serve warm with additional berries, maple syrup (optional), and a sprinkle of chopped nuts if desired.

Label: High in fiber and whole grains, good source of protein, customizable with different fruits and toppings, gluten-free option (use gluten-free flour blend).

Berry Almond Smoothie Bowl

Ingredients:

- 1/2 cup mixed frozen berries
- 1/2 banana, frozen
- 1/2 cup plain Greek yogurt (low-fat or unsweetened almond milk option)
- 1/4 cup unsweetened almond milk
- 1/4 cup rolled oats
- 1 tablespoon almond butter
- 1/4 teaspoon vanilla extract
- Dash of ground cinnamon
- Optional toppings: fresh berries, chopped nuts, granola, chia seeds

Nutritional Information (per serving):

- Calories: 350
- Fat: 10g (2g saturated)
- Carbs: 40g (5g fiber)
- Protein: 15g
- Calcium: 300mg (30% DV)

Cooking Time: 5 minutes

Serving size: 1

Instructions:

1. Blend frozen berries, bananas, yogurt, almond milk, and oats until smooth and creamy.
2. Pour into a bowl and top with almond butter, vanilla extract, and cinnamon.
3. Get creative with additional toppings like fresh berries, chopped nuts, granola, or chia seeds for added texture and flavor.

Label: Rich in protein and calcium, good source of healthy fats and fiber, customizable with different fruits and toppings, vegan option (use plant-based yogurt and milk).

Yogurt-Covered Frozen Grapes

Ingredients:

- 1 cup green or red grapes, washed and patted dry
- 1/2 cup plain Greek yogurt (low-fat or unsweetened almond milk option)
- 1/4 cup chopped almonds or pistachios
- Honey or maple syrup drizzle (optional)

Nutritional Information (per serving):

- Calories: 200
- Fat: 5g (1g saturated)
- Carbs: 35g (3g fiber)
- Protein: 10g
- Calcium: 200mg (20% DV)

Cooking Time: 10 minutes (plus freezing time)

Serving size: 1

Instructions:

1. Line a baking sheet with parchment paper.
2. Dip each grape into the yogurt, coating it evenly.
3. Place coated grapes on the prepared baking sheet and sprinkle with chopped nuts.
4. Put it in the freezer for at least 2 hours or until it becomes hard.
5. Drizzle with honey or maple syrup (optional) before serving.

Label: Low-calorie and refreshing, good source of protein and calcium, perfect for a sweet treat, dairy-free option (use plant-based yogurt).

Lunch Recipes

Grilled Chicken Caesar Salad

Ingredients:

- 4 ounces boneless, skinless chicken breast
- 2 cups romaine lettuce, chopped
- 1/4 cup cherry tomatoes, halved
- 1/4 cup grated Parmesan cheese
- 2 tablespoons Caesar dressing (low-fat option encouraged)
- 1/4 cup whole-wheat croutons (optional)
- Olive oil for grilling
- Salt and pepper to taste

Cooking Time: 15 minutes

Serving size: 1

Instructions:

1. Before cooking, warm up the grill to medium heat. Put olive oil on the chicken, and sprinkle it with salt and pepper. Grill each side for 5-7 minutes until it's fully cooked.
2. While the chicken cooks, prepare salad by combining romaine lettuce, cherry tomatoes, and Parmesan cheese in a bowl.
3. Slice grilled chicken and add it to the salad.
4. Drizzle with Caesar dressing and toss gently to combine.
5. Top with whole-wheat croutons (optional) and enjoy!

Nutritional Information (per serving):

- Calories: 350
- Fat: 15g (3g saturated)
- Carbs: 15g (3g fiber)
- Protein: 35g
- Calcium: 200mg (20% DV)

Tuna and White Bean Salad

Ingredients:

- 1 (12-ounce) can of tuna, packed in water, drained, and flaked
- 1 (15-ounce) can cannellini beans, rinsed and drained
- 1/2 cup chopped cucumber
- 1/4 cup chopped red onion
- 1/4 cup chopped celery
- 2 tablespoons chopped fresh parsley
- 1 tablespoon olive oil
- 2 tablespoons lemon juice
- 1/2 teaspoon Dijon mustard
- Salt and pepper to taste

Cooking Time: 10 minutes

Serving size: 2

Instructions:

1. Combine tuna, cannellini beans, cucumber, red onion, celery, and parsley in a bowl.
2. In another bowl, mix olive oil, lemon juice, and Dijon mustard. Pour this dressing on the salad and mix everything.
3. Season with salt and pepper to taste.
4. Serve on whole-wheat bread or as a salad with lettuce leaves (optional).

Nutritional Information (per serving):

- Calories: 300
- Fat: 5g (1g saturated)
- Carbs: 30g (5g fiber)
- Protein: 25g
- Calcium: 100mg (10% DV)

Lentil and Spinach Dal'

Ingredients:

- 1 cup brown lentils, rinsed
- 4 cups vegetable broth (low-sodium preferred)
- 1 tablespoon olive oil
- 1 onion, chopped
- 2 cloves garlic, minced
- 1 inch fresh ginger, grated
- 1 teaspoon ground cumin
- 1/2 teaspoon ground coriander
- 1/4 teaspoon red chili flakes (optional)
- 1 (15-ounce) can diced tomatoes, undrained
- 5 cups fresh spinach
- 1/4 cup plain Greek yogurt (low-fat or plant-based alternative)
- Salt and pepper to taste

Cooking Time: 30 minutes

Serving size: 4

Instructions:

1. In a pot, combine lentils and vegetable broth. Bring to a boil, then reduce heat and simmer for 20 minutes, or until lentils are tender.
2. While waiting, warm up olive oil in a pan on medium heat. Put onions in and cook until they become soft, which takes about 5 minutes.
3. Add garlic, ginger, cumin, coriander, and red chili flakes (if using). Cook for 1 minute until fragrant.
4. Stir in diced tomatoes and cook for 5 minutes more.
5. Add the tomato mixture and spinach to the pot with cooked lentils. Simmer for 5 minutes, or until spinach is wilted.
6. Mix in Greek yogurt and add salt and pepper to taste.

Nutritional Information (per serving):

- Calories: 250
- Fat: 5g (1g saturated)
- Carbs: 40g (8g fiber)
- Protein: 15g
- Calcium: 150mg (15% DV)

Turkey and Vegetable Stir-Fry

Ingredients:

- 1 tablespoon vegetable oil
- One pound of turkey breast without bones or skin sliced thinly.
- 1 red bell pepper, sliced
- 1 green bell pepper, sliced
- 1 broccoli floret, cut into bite-sized pieces
- 1 carrot, julienned
- 1/2 cup sugar snap peas
- 1/4 cup green onions, chopped
- 2 tablespoons low-sodium soy sauce
- 1 tablespoon rice vinegar
- 1 tablespoon cornstarch
- 1/2 teaspoon grated ginger
- 1/4 teaspoon red pepper flakes (optional)
- Cooked brown rice or quinoa (for serving)

Nutritional Information (per serving):

- Calories: 350
- Fat: 10g (2g saturated)
- Carbs: 40g (5g fiber)
- Protein: 30g
- Calcium: 100mg (10% DV)

Cooking Time: 15 minutes

Serving size: 2

Instructions:

1. Warm up oil in a big skillet or wok on medium-high heat. Put in the turkey and cook until it turns brown, which usually takes about 5 minutes. Take it out of the pan and set it aside.
2. Add bell peppers, broccoli, and carrot to the pan and stir-fry for 3-4 minutes, until slightly softened.
3. Stir in sugar snap peas and cook for 1 minute more.
4. In a small bowl, whisk together soy sauce, rice vinegar, cornstarch, ginger, and red pepper flakes (if using).
5. Return the turkey to the pan and pour in the sauce. Stir-fry for 1-2 minutes, until sauce thickens slightly.
6. Garnish with chopped green onions and serve over cooked brown rice or quinoa.

Label: High in protein and vegetables, good source of fiber and vitamins, customizable with different vegetables and spices, gluten-free option (use rice noodle alternative).

Miso-Glazed Cod

Ingredients:

- 1 cod fillet (4-6 ounces)
- 2 tablespoons miso paste
- 1 tablespoon honey
- 1 tablespoon mirin (sweet cooking wine)
- 1 tablespoon rice vinegar
- 1 tablespoon water
- 1 teaspoon fresh ginger, grated
- 1/2 teaspoon sesame oil
- 1/4 cup chopped green onions
- Cooked brown rice or quinoa (for serving)

Nutritional Information (per serving):

- Calories: 300
- Fat: 10g (2g saturated)
- Carbs: 30g (4g fiber)
- Protein: 35g
- Calcium: 70mg (7% DV)

Cooking Time: 15 minutes

Serving size: 1

Instructions:

1. Preheat the oven to 400°F (200°C).
2. In a small bowl, whisk together miso paste, honey, mirin, rice vinegar, water, ginger, and sesame oil.
3. Place cod fillet in a baking dish and brush with half of the miso glaze.
4. Put it in the oven and bake for 10-12 minutes, or until it's fully cooked.
5. While cod cooks, prepare brown rice or quinoa.
6. Baste cod with remaining glaze before serving. Garnish with chopped green onions and serve over brown rice or quinoa.

Label: Rich in protein and omega-3 fatty acids, flavorful and easy to prepare, gluten-free and dairy-free option (use vegan miso paste).

Sardine and Avocado Sandwich

Ingredients:

- 2 slices whole-wheat bread
- 1/2 ripe avocado, thinly sliced
- 4 canned sardines, drained and packed in water (bone-in or boneless)
- 1 tablespoon lemon juice
- 1/4 teaspoon Dijon mustard
- Pinch of salt and pepper
- Handful of mixed greens (optional)

Nutritional Information (per serving):

- Calories: 300
- Fat: 20g (3g saturated)
- Carbs: 35g (5g fiber)
- Protein: 25g
- Calcium: 180mg (18% DV)

Cooking Time: 5 minutes

Serving size: 1

Instructions:

1. Mash avocado slices with lemon juice, Dijon mustard, salt, and pepper.
2. Toast bread and spread with the avocado mixture.
3. Top each slice with sardines.
4. Add mixed greens (optional) for extra flavor and nutrients.

Label: High in protein and omega-3 fatty acids, healthy fat source, quick and easy lunch option. Rich in calcium and vitamin D, perfect for bone health, a light and refreshing sandwich.

Dinner Recipes

Creamy Broccoli and Cheddar Soup

Ingredients:

- 1 tablespoon olive oil
- 1 onion, chopped
- 2 cloves garlic, minced
- 4 cups vegetable broth (low-sodium preferred)
- 3 cups chopped broccoli florets
- 1/2 cup chopped potato (optional, for thickening)
- 1/2 cup heavy cream (low-fat or unsweetened almond milk alternative)
- 1 cup grated cheddar cheese
- 1/4 teaspoon ground nutmeg
- Salt and pepper to taste

|Osteoporosis Diet Cookbook for Seniors|

Nutritional Information (per serving):

- Calories: 250 (based on using low-fat options)
- Fat: 10g (4g saturated)
- Carbs: 25g (4g fiber)
- Protein: 15g
- Calcium: 300mg (30% DV)

Cooking Time: 20 minutes

Serving size: 4-5

Instructions:

1. Warm up olive oil in a big pot on medium heat. Put in onions and cook until they become soft, around 5 minutes. Add garlic and cook for an additional minute. Pour in vegetable broth and bring it to a boil. Add broccoli and potato (if using) and let it simmer for 10 minutes, or until the veggies are tender.
2. Puree soup using an immersion blender or in batches in a regular blender until smooth.
3. Return the soup to the pot and stir in heavy cream or milk alternative, cheddar cheese,

and nutmeg. Add salt and pepper to your liking.
4. Heat through until warmed through, but do not boil.
5. Serve hot, garnished with additional grated cheese or chopped fresh herbs (optional).

Label: High in calcium and vitamin C, creamy comfort food made healthy, customizable with different vegetables and spices, gluten-free option (use gluten-free bread for dipping).

Baked Salmon with Dill and Lemon

Ingredients:

- 2 salmon fillets (4-6 ounces each)
- 1 tablespoon olive oil
- 1 tablespoon lemon juice
- 1/2 teaspoon dried dill
- 1/4 teaspoon salt
- 1/4 teaspoon black pepper
- 1 lemon, sliced (optional)

Nutritional Information (per serving):

- Calories: 350
- Fat: 15g (2g saturated)
- Carbs: 2g
- Protein: 40g
- Calcium: 50mg (5% DV)

Cooking Time: 15 minutes

Serving size: 2

Instructions:

1. Preheat the oven to 400°F (200°C). Line a baking sheet with parchment paper.
2. In a tiny bowl, mix olive oil, lemon juice, dill, salt, and pepper using a whisk.
3. Brush the salmon fillets with the mixture and place on the prepared baking sheet.
4. Top with lemon slices (optional).
5. Put it in the oven and bake for 10-15 minutes, or until the salmon is fully cooked and easily flakes when prodded with a fork. Pair it with roasted vegetables or a side salad for a wholesome meal.

Label: Rich in protein and omega-3 fatty acids, this light and flavorful dish, is easy to prepare, and oven-safe for seniors.

Spinach and Feta Stuffed Chicken Breast

Ingredients:

- 4 boneless, skinless chicken breasts
- 1 tablespoon olive oil
- 1/2 onion, chopped
- 2 cloves garlic, minced
- Use 10 ounces of frozen spinach, thaw it, and squeeze out the excess water.
- 1/2 cup crumbled feta cheese
- 1/4 cup chopped fresh parsley
- 1/4 teaspoon dried oregano
- Salt and pepper to taste
- 1/4 cup chicken broth (optional)

Nutritional Information (per serving):

- Calories: 300
- Fat: 10g (3g saturated)
- Carbs: 5g
- Protein: 40g
- Calcium: 180mg (18% DV)

Cooking Time: 30 minutes

Serving size: 4

Instructions:

1. Preheat the oven to 400°F (200°C).
2. Butterfly each chicken breast by carefully slicing it open horizontally, not cutting it all the way through. Open the chicken like a book.
3. Warm up olive oil in a pan on medium heat. Put in onions and cook until they become soft approximately 5 minutes. Then, add garlic and cook for an additional minute.
4. Stir in spinach, feta cheese, parsley, and oregano. Season with salt and pepper to taste. Cook until spinach is wilted and mixture thickens slightly about 2-3 minutes. Remove from heat.
5. Divide the spinach mixture evenly between the open chicken breasts. Spread it out to form a thin layer. Roll up the chicken breasts tightly, securing them with toothpicks if necessary.
6. Place rolled chicken breasts seam-side down in a baking dish. Pour in 1/4 cup chicken broth (optional) for added moisture.
7. Bake for 20-25 minutes, or until chicken is cooked through and juices run clear when pierced with a fork.
8. Serve hot with roasted vegetables or a side salad for a complete and nutritious meal.

Label: High in protein and calcium, flavorful and filling, healthy alternative to fried chicken, gluten-free option (use gluten-free breading if desired).

Quinoa and Black Bean Stuffed Peppers

Ingredients:

- 4 bell peppers (red, yellow, or orange)
- 1 cup quinoa, rinsed
- 15-ounce can of black beans, drain them, and give them a good rinse.
- 1/2 cup chopped onion
- 1 clove garlic, minced
- 1 cup diced tomatoes (fresh or canned)
- 1/2 cup corn kernels
- 1/4 cup chopped fresh cilantro
- 1 tablespoon olive oil
- 1/2 teaspoon cumin
- 1/4 teaspoon chili powder
- Salt and pepper to taste
- Optional toppings: shredded cheese, avocado slices, sour cream

Nutritional Information (per serving):

- Calories: 350
- Fat: 5g (1g saturated)
- Carbs: 45g (5g fiber)
- Protein: 15g
- Calcium: 100mg (10% DV)

Cooking Time: 40 minutes

Serving size: 4

Instructions:

1. Preheat the oven to 400°F (200°C). Line a baking dish with parchment paper.
2. Cook quinoa according to package instructions.
3. While the quinoa cooks, prepare the filling. Warm up olive oil in a skillet over medium heat. Put in onions and cook until they become soft, around 5 minutes. Then, add garlic, cumin, and chili powder, and cook for an extra minute until it smells aromatic.
4. Stir in black beans, tomatoes, corn, and cilantro. Season with salt and pepper to taste. Let it cook for 5 minutes until it's warm all the way through.
5. Once quinoa is cooked, fluff it with a fork and stir it into the bean mixture.
6. Cut the tops off the bell peppers and discard or reserve for garnish. Remove seeds and membranes.
7. Fill each pepper with the quinoa mixture, packing it loosely.

8. Place stuffed peppers in the prepared baking dish. Cover with foil and bake for 20-25 minutes, or until peppers are tender.
9. Serve hot with desired toppings.

Label: High in fiber and plant-based protein, customizable with different vegetables and spices, gluten-free and vegan options (skip cheese and sour cream).

Beef and Barley Vegetable Soup

Ingredients:

- 1 tablespoon olive oil
- 1 pound lean ground beef (90% lean or turkey can be substituted)
- 1 onion, chopped
- 2 carrots, chopped
- 2 celery stalks, chopped
- 2 cloves garlic, minced
- 8 cups low-sodium beef broth
- 1 cup barley, rinsed
- 4 cups chopped vegetables (such as potatoes, green beans, broccoli, carrots)
- 1 (14.5-ounce) can of diced tomatoes, undrained
- 1 teaspoon dried thyme
- 1/2 teaspoon dried oregano
- Salt and pepper to taste

Nutritional Information (per serving):

- Calories: 300
- Fat: 10g (3g saturated)
- Carbs: 35g (5g fiber)
- Protein: 25g
- Calcium: 50mg (5% DV)

Cooking Time: 45 minutes

Serving size: 6

Instructions:

1. In a large saucepan, heat the olive oil over medium heat. Cook until the ground beef is browned, breaking it up with a spoon.
2. Remove any extra fat.
3. Cook until the onion, carrots, and celery are cooked, about 5 minutes.
4. Combine the garlic, beef broth, barley, and chopped veggies in a mixing bowl. Bring to a boil, then lower to a low heat and continue to cook for 30 minutes, or until the barley is soft.
5. Add the diced tomatoes, thyme, and oregano and mix well. Season to taste with salt and pepper.
6. Simmer for another 10 minutes, or until well cooked.
7. Serve hot with crusty bread or rolls.

Label: Hearty and comforting soup, a good source of protein and fiber, customizable with different vegetables and spices, gluten-free option (use gluten-free barley alternative).

Roast Pork Tenderloin with Apples

Ingredients:

- 1 (1-1.5 pound) pork tenderloin
- 2 tablespoons olive oil
- 1/2 teaspoon dried thyme
- 1/2 teaspoon salt
- 1/4 teaspoon black pepper
- 2 apples (crisp varieties like Granny Smith or Honeycrisp), cored and sliced
- 1/2 cup chicken broth
- 1 tablespoon honey
- 1 tablespoon Dijon mustard
- Optional garnish: fresh thyme sprigs, chopped parsley

Nutritional Information (per serving):

- Calories: 350
- Fat: 15g (3g saturated)
- Carbs: 25g (3g fiber)
- Protein: 35g
- Calcium: 50mg (5% DV)

Cooking Time: 30 minutes

Serving size: 4

Instructions:

1. Preheat the oven to 400°F (200°C). Line a baking dish with parchment paper.
2. Pat the pork tenderloin dry with paper towels. Rub with olive oil, thyme, salt, and pepper.
3. Toss apple slices with 1 tablespoon of olive oil and arrange around the pork tenderloin in the prepared baking dish.
4. In a small bowl, whisk together chicken broth, honey, and Dijon mustard. Pour over the pork and apples.
5. Roast for 20-25 minutes, or until the pork is cooked through and reaches an internal temperature of 145°F (63°C).
6. Baste the pork and apples with pan juices during the last 5 minutes of cooking.
7. Let the pork rest for 5 minutes before slicing.
8. Serve pork sliced with roasted apples and drizzled with pan juices. Garnish with fresh thyme sprigs or chopped parsley, if desired.

Label: Lean protein source, sweet and savory combination, customizable with different fruits and vegetables, gluten-free option (use gluten-free broth and mustard).

Greek-Style Baked Eggplant

Ingredients:

- 2 medium eggplants
- 2 tablespoons olive oil
- 1/2 teaspoon dried oregano
- 1/2 teaspoon salt
- 1/4 teaspoon black pepper
- 4 tomatoes, thinly sliced
- 1/2 red onion, thinly sliced
- 1/4 cup crumbled feta cheese
- 2 tablespoons chopped fresh parsley
- 2 tablespoons balsamic vinegar (optional)

Nutritional Information (per serving):

- Calories: 250
- Fat: 10g (2g saturated)
- Carbs: 25g (5g fiber)
- Protein: 10g
- Calcium: 150mg (15% DV)

Cooking Time: 45 minutes

Serving size: 4

Instructions:

1. Preheat the oven to 400°F (200°C). Line a baking sheet with parchment paper.
2. Cut eggplants in half lengthwise. Scoop out the flesh, leaving a 1/2-inch border. Dice the flesh.
3. Drizzle the eggplant halves with olive oil and season with oregano, salt, and pepper.
4. Place the eggplant halves on the prepared baking sheet and bake for 20 minutes.
5. Meanwhile, heat 1 tablespoon of olive oil in a pan over medium heat. Add chopped eggplant flesh and cook until softened about 5 minutes.
6. Stir in tomatoes, red onion, salt, and pepper. Cook for an additional 5 minutes, until tomatoes are slightly softened.
7. Fill the baked eggplant halves with the tomato mixture. Top with crumbled feta cheese and parsley.
8. Drizzle with balsamic vinegar (optional) and bake for an additional 10-15 minutes, until heated through and feta cheese is melted.
9. Serve immediately with fresh bread and a side salad.

Label: Low-calorie vegetarian option, a good source of vitamins and antioxidants, customizable with different herbs and spices, gluten-free and vegan option (skip feta cheese).

Turkey and Kale Stuffed Acorn Squash

Ingredients:

- 2 acorn squash (medium-sized)
- 1 tablespoon olive oil
- 1/2 teaspoon salt
- 1/4 teaspoon black pepper
- 1 pound ground turkey (90% lean)
- 1 onion, chopped
- 2 cloves garlic, minced
- 4 cups chopped kale (massaged)
- 1/2 cup chopped mushrooms (optional)
- 1/2 cup cooked brown rice (optional)
- 1/4 cup chicken broth
- 1/4 cup chopped fresh parsley
- 1/4 cup grated Parmesan cheese (optional)

Nutritional Information (per serving):

- Calories: 400
- Fat: 15g (3g saturated)
- Carbs: 35g (6g fiber)
- Protein: 35g
- Calcium: 100mg (10% DV)

Cooking Time: 45 minutes

Serving size: 4

Instructions:

1. Preheat the oven to 400°F (200°C). Line a baking sheet with parchment paper.
2. Cut the acorn squash in half lengthwise and scoop out the seeds and membranes. Drizzle with olive oil, season with salt and pepper, and place cut-side down on the prepared baking sheet.
3. Bake for 20 minutes, or until the squash is softened and slightly tender.
4. In a large pan over medium heat, heat the olive oil while the squash cooks. Cook until the ground turkey is browned, breaking it up with a spoon. Remove any extra fat.

5. Cook until the onion is softened, approximately 5 minutes.
6. Cook for 1 minute more after adding the garlic.
7. Add kale and cook, stirring occasionally, until wilted and softened, about 5 minutes. Add mushrooms if using.
8. Stir in cooked brown rice (optional), chicken broth, and parsley. Season to taste with salt and pepper.
9. Once the squash is cooked, turn it right-side up. Fill each half with the turkey and kale mixture, packing it loosely.
10. Sprinkle with Parmesan cheese (optional) and bake for an additional 15-20 minutes, or until heated through and bubbly.
11. Serve hot, with a side of roasted vegetables or a salad for a complete meal.

Label: High in protein and fiber, rich in vitamins and minerals, customizable with different vegetables and herbs, gluten-free and dairy-free option (skip brown rice and Parmesan cheese).

Conclusion

You've concluded this cookbook, but not the end of your adventure. You've learned how to eat healthy and keep your bones strong by following the recipes and ideas in this book. You've also learned to appreciate your cuisine and your life by sharing your tales and experiences with others you care about. But there is always more to learn and explore. Several additional meals and recipes may replenish both your bones and your spirit. There are several ways to adjust and personalize the recipes in this book to fit your interests and needs. Using your imagination and inventiveness, you may design your recipes and stories. So don't stop here. Continue cooking, eating, and living. Continue to experience new flavors and adventures. Maintain your health and pleasure. Keep inspiring and being inspired by others. Most essential, keep smiling and glowing. You are a star, and you deserve to shine. Thank you for selecting this cookbook. I hope you appreciated it as much as I did. I hope you found it informative and beneficial. I hope you will return to it again and again. Until next time, bon appetit and happy cooking!

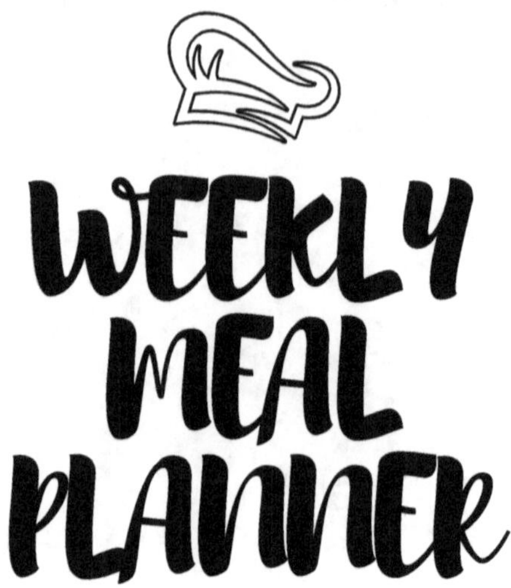

WEEKLY MEAL PLANNER

WEEKLY MEAL PLANNER

SUNDAY	BREAKFAST	
	LUNCH	
	DINNER	
MONDAY	BREAKFAST	
	LUNCH	
	DINNER	
TUESDAY	BREAKFAST	
	LUNCH	
	DINNER	
WEDNESDAY	BREAKFAST	
	LUNCH	
	DINNER	
THURSDAY	BREAKFAST	
	LUNCH	
	DINNER	
FRIDAY	BREAKFAST	
	LUNCH	
	DINNER	
SATURDAY	BREAKFAST	
	LUNCH	
	DINNER	

GROCERY LIST

SNACKS

WEEKLY MEAL PLANNER

SUNDAY	BREAKFAST	
	LUNCH	
	DINNER	
MONDAY	BREAKFAST	
	LUNCH	
	DINNER	
TUESDAY	BREAKFAST	
	LUNCH	
	DINNER	
WEDNESDAY	BREAKFAST	
	LUNCH	
	DINNER	
THURSDAY	BREAKFAST	
	LUNCH	
	DINNER	
FRIDAY	BREAKFAST	
	LUNCH	
	DINNER	
SATURDAY	BREAKFAST	
	LUNCH	
	DINNER	

GROCERY LIST

SNACKS

WEEKLY MEAL PLANNER

SUNDAY	BREAKFAST	
	LUNCH	
	DINNER	
MONDAY	BREAKFAST	
	LUNCH	
	DINNER	
TUESDAY	BREAKFAST	
	LUNCH	
	DINNER	
WEDNESDAY	BREAKFAST	
	LUNCH	
	DINNER	
THURSDAY	BREAKFAST	
	LUNCH	
	DINNER	
FRIDAY	BREAKFAST	
	LUNCH	
	DINNER	
SATURDAY	BREAKFAST	
	LUNCH	
	DINNER	

GROCERY LIST

SNACKS

WEEKLY MEAL PLANNER

SUNDAY	BREAKFAST	
	LUNCH	
	DINNER	
MONDAY	BREAKFAST	
	LUNCH	
	DINNER	
TUESDAY	BREAKFAST	
	LUNCH	
	DINNER	
WEDNESDAY	BREAKFAST	
	LUNCH	
	DINNER	
THURSDAY	BREAKFAST	
	LUNCH	
	DINNER	
FRIDAY	BREAKFAST	
	LUNCH	
	DINNER	
SATURDAY	BREAKFAST	
	LUNCH	
	DINNER	

GROCERY LIST

SNACKS

WEEKLY MEAL PLANNER

SUNDAY		
	BREAKFAST	
	LUNCH	
	DINNER	

MONDAY		
	BREAKFAST	
	LUNCH	
	DINNER	

TUESDAY		
	BREAKFAST	
	LUNCH	
	DINNER	

WEDNESDAY		
	BREAKFAST	
	LUNCH	
	DINNER	

THURSDAY		
	BREAKFAST	
	LUNCH	
	DINNER	

FRIDAY		
	BREAKFAST	
	LUNCH	
	DINNER	

SATURDAY		
	BREAKFAST	
	LUNCH	
	DINNER	

GROCERY LIST

SNACKS

WEEKLY MEAL PLANNER

SUNDAY	BREAKFAST	
	LUNCH	
	DINNER	
MONDAY	BREAKFAST	
	LUNCH	
	DINNER	
TUESDAY	BREAKFAST	
	LUNCH	
	DINNER	
WEDNESDAY	BREAKFAST	
	LUNCH	
	DINNER	
THURSDAY	BREAKFAST	
	LUNCH	
	DINNER	
FRIDAY	BREAKFAST	
	LUNCH	
	DINNER	
SATURDAY	BREAKFAST	
	LUNCH	
	DINNER	

GROCERY LIST

SNACKS

WEEKLY MEAL PLANNER

SUNDAY	BREAKFAST	
	LUNCH	
	DINNER	
MONDAY	BREAKFAST	
	LUNCH	
	DINNER	
TUESDAY	BREAKFAST	
	LUNCH	
	DINNER	
WEDNESDAY	BREAKFAST	
	LUNCH	
	DINNER	
THURSDAY	BREAKFAST	
	LUNCH	
	DINNER	
FRIDAY	BREAKFAST	
	LUNCH	
	DINNER	
SATURDAY	BREAKFAST	
	LUNCH	
	DINNER	

GROCERY LIST

SNACKS

WEEKLY MEAL PLANNER

SUNDAY	BREAKFAST	
	LUNCH	
	DINNER	

MONDAY	BREAKFAST	
	LUNCH	
	DINNER	

TUESDAY	BREAKFAST	
	LUNCH	
	DINNER	

WEDNESDAY	BREAKFAST	
	LUNCH	
	DINNER	

THURSDAY	BREAKFAST	
	LUNCH	
	DINNER	

FRIDAY	BREAKFAST	
	LUNCH	
	DINNER	

SATURDAY	BREAKFAST	
	LUNCH	
	DINNER	

GROCERY LIST

SNACKS

WEEKLY MEAL PLANNER

SUNDAY	BREAKFAST	
	LUNCH	
	DINNER	
MONDAY	BREAKFAST	
	LUNCH	
	DINNER	
TUESDAY	BREAKFAST	
	LUNCH	
	DINNER	
WEDNESDAY	BREAKFAST	
	LUNCH	
	DINNER	
THURSDAY	BREAKFAST	
	LUNCH	
	DINNER	
FRIDAY	BREAKFAST	
	LUNCH	
	DINNER	
SATURDAY	BREAKFAST	
	LUNCH	
	DINNER	

GROCERY LIST

SNACKS

WEEKLY MEAL PLANNER

SUNDAY	BREAKFAST	
	LUNCH	
	DINNER	

MONDAY	BREAKFAST	
	LUNCH	
	DINNER	

TUESDAY	BREAKFAST	
	LUNCH	
	DINNER	

WEDNESDAY	BREAKFAST	
	LUNCH	
	DINNER	

THURSDAY	BREAKFAST	
	LUNCH	
	DINNER	

FRIDAY	BREAKFAST	
	LUNCH	
	DINNER	

SATURDAY	BREAKFAST	
	LUNCH	
	DINNER	

GROCERY LIST

SNACKS

WEEKLY MEAL PLANNER

SUNDAY	BREAKFAST	
	LUNCH	
	DINNER	
MONDAY	BREAKFAST	
	LUNCH	
	DINNER	
TUESDAY	BREAKFAST	
	LUNCH	
	DINNER	
WEDNESDAY	BREAKFAST	
	LUNCH	
	DINNER	
THURSDAY	BREAKFAST	
	LUNCH	
	DINNER	
FRIDAY	BREAKFAST	
	LUNCH	
	DINNER	
SATURDAY	BREAKFAST	
	LUNCH	
	DINNER	

GROCERY LIST

SNACKS

WEEKLY MEAL PLANNER

SUNDAY	BREAKFAST	
	LUNCH	
	DINNER	
MONDAY	BREAKFAST	
	LUNCH	
	DINNER	
TUESDAY	BREAKFAST	
	LUNCH	
	DINNER	
WEDNESDAY	BREAKFAST	
	LUNCH	
	DINNER	
THURSDAY	BREAKFAST	
	LUNCH	
	DINNER	
FRIDAY	BREAKFAST	
	LUNCH	
	DINNER	
SATURDAY	BREAKFAST	
	LUNCH	
	DINNER	

GROCERY LIST

SNACKS